PORN vs. Prayer

GRAYDON MCINTYRE

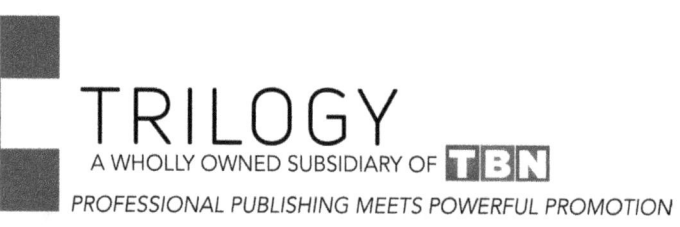

Trilogy Christian Publishers
A Wholly Owned Subsidiary of Trinity Broadcasting Network
2442 Michelle Drive
Tustin, CA 92780
Copyright © 2024 by Graydon McIntyre
All Scripture quotations, unless otherwise noted, taken from Revised Standard Version of the Bible, copyright 1952 by the Division of Christian Education of the National Council of the Churches of Christ in the United States of America. All rights reserved.
All rights reserved, including the right to reproduce this book or portions thereof in any form whatsoever.
For information, address Trilogy Christian Publishing
Rights Department, 2442 Michelle Drive, Tustin, CA 92780.
Trilogy Christian Publishing/ TBN and colophon are trademarks of Trinity Broadcasting Network.
For information about special discounts for bulk purchases, please contact Trilogy Christian Publishing.

Trilogy Disclaimer: The views and content expressed in this book are those of the author and may not necessarily reflect the views and doctrine of Trilogy Christian Publishing or the Trinity Broadcasting Network.

10 9 8 7 6 5 4 3 2 1
Library of Congress Cataloging-in-Publication Data is available.
ISBN 979-8-89041-909-5
ISBN 979-8-89041-910-1 (ebook)

Dedication

To God the Father, God the Son, and God the Spirit.

May this book serve not my will but yours.

Forward

It was not my idea to write this book and, to be honest, I would never have conceptualized writing it if God didn't ask this of me. At the beginning of 2023, someone in my church thought I would be a good fit for a more active role. At that point, I wasn't even a confirmed Catholic yet and in faith reformation. I made every excuse I could think of to disqualify myself. All they said is God doesn't call the qualified, He qualifies the called. Instead of making more excuses I reflected and tried to think about what God might be calling me to do. As it turned out, the mission I had in mind had more steps than initially realized, so I decided to be patient and wait. On the night of the Easter Vigil, after weeks of waiting, I became impatient waiting on God. After the vigil ended, before I went to sleep, I prayed to God, telling Him what I was working on and that I knew that He was working on it with me. Then I asked Him what I should do while I waited, then a voice in my head said, "Why don't you write a book about your experiences with porn and how you quit." So here I am writing a book about my experiences with porn and how I quit.

Table of Contents

Dedication 5

Forward 7

Prologue 11

   1: The Truth About Porn 15

   2: Rules, Tips 'n' Tricks 21

   3: What to Expect 43

Epilogue 53

Bibliography 55

Prologue

Since you've opened this book it's safe to assume one of the following:

A. You are trying to quit and can't seem to shake it off.

B. You were clean for a while then relapsed and now question if you'll ever be able to break free from pornography.

C. You have tried every practical thing you can and are willing to try anything to eliminate your addiction.

The good news is by picking this up you are acknowledging that you are struggling to quit porn for whatever reason. Maybe you thought it was something innocent until you realized how dangerous it is, that you could stop at any time- and were wrong.

Like other addictions, the brain rewired itself to prioritize the addiction.

Unlike other addictions, the source doesn't come from external stimuli. This addiction is sourced and sustained in your brain. The more you participate in watching porn or looking at an image or person with sexual intent, the stronger and more potent the addiction becomes.

Unlike alcohol and drugs, it's impossible to avoid.

PRAYER VS PORN

The majority of pop culture is sexuality based: you hear it in music, see it in movies, and it is plastered all over the internet—you can't escape it. Social media features sex workers labeled as "influencers" and promote them as cultural focuses. That's just part of living in the modern day. Most people, especially young men, grow up in a hypersexualized world under the influence of pornography—myself included.

I was exposed to pornography as far back as I can remember. My father was a porn addict. This was only intensified by his seclusion. Half the time, when I would walk into his office, he'd quickly be minimizing chat room tabs or a porn video he was watching. Saturday mornings were TV shows featuring either close-up practically nude women posing on a beach, or wild drunk girls, which usually lead to stripping or worse. Somewhere between eight and nine, I noticed that I got excited from the shows my dad watched, and curious why, I looked into it myself. The next thing I knew I was thirteen years old masturbating between three to five times per day. I knew I had to stop. I could see how it affected my life, and that my inactivity only worsened it. I tried to quit several times but failed each time. This went on for years. Eventually, I gave up on the idea of getting clean.

At the beginning of 2020, everything changed, as I'm sure it did for all of you when the COVID-19 quarantine started. Then, I was interning at a company and delivered food on the side. Well, in reality, I delivered food full time

PROLOGUE

and was an intern on the side. So when the quarantine started, I did what everyone else did—I played video games all day and intermittently got bored, so that turned into watching porn all day.

After about a month in quarantine, my dad called me. Preoccupied with video games, I wasn't attentive during the phone call. He asked about work, and I mumbled that everyone was in quarantine so I couldn't work. Then he asked me, "Son, what are you doing? You're not working, you're not going to school. Are you going to do anything with your life or are you just going to sit on the couch and do nothing?" Those words infuriated me, and when I reflected on why, I realized he was right. I wasn't where I wanted to be in life. I thought about everything I hated about myself: I was fat, in a dead-end delivery job, and overall miserable. When I looked into what caused my misery, porn was the biggest culprit.

I knew from all my failed attempts at quitting, I was not disciplined enough to break my porn habits, but I decided I could do something about my weight. I started small, portioning what I ate. When the gyms opened up, I went. I adjusted old high school workouts to what I could practically maintain. In the meantime, I doubled down in my delivery job and the internship. This allowed me to quit my delivery job to focus on my internship and pursue my dream career. This was not immediate; it took me almost a year to get to this point. But I wasn't done making life changes. I started going to church again and joined the young adult group.

After 8 months of successfully fighting pornography, I relapsed. Instead of falling into despair and giving up, I researched porn addictions, as well as addictions as a whole. At first, I followed practical advice. this helped but wasn't the answer. I'd still feel overwhelming urges prodding and goading me to watch porn. It felt like someone was in my head flashing pornographic images, trying to overpower me. So I tried something new. I prayed to God to remove this temptation from me. And He did. As I prayed more often, I was less tempted. Even the overwhelming urges became easier to subdue, passing quicker than before I had tried praying.

    I had struggled for over a decade with pornography and the guilt, shame, and regret that comes with it. Learn from my mistakes- learn what works, and to some extent why, and break free from the chains of pornography to live free, joyful, and peaceful lives. Nothing about this is easy. Many of you also started watching porn pre-pubescently and will have to undo years of conditioning. You might even find that porn causes you to struggle with normal, organic relationships. This is normal because the false interpretation of the correlation between sex and relationships porn engrains in you. We'll go over the true purpose of relationships and how healthy relationships function after breaking free from porn.

1

The Truth About Porn

Let's start with the simple truth: porn isn't real. It's written, scripted, edited, and produced to make money. Plain and simple. And like any other industry, it wants to make more money, so companies make more porn to upstage their competitors, which contributed to porn becoming the aggressive, domineering, and objectifying videos that exist now.

Every part of pornography is intentional—the lighting, color schemes, facial expressions, all of it. Just to increase the chance you'll watch their videos, and better yet—pay to access what is behind their paywall. This is just their business, but it is your life.

Why is porn so addictive? It hijacks the natural desire to reproduce. It stimulates and creates arousal, and with continual and perpetual consumption, the brain becomes numb to any other stimulus. And, just like that, addiction. Porn is the most common outlet, but even masturbation alone can create similar effects.

We are biologically driven, as living creatures, to reproduce and carry our genes to the next generation. Porn takes advantage of this, playing into the primal part of the human brain that generates sexual satisfaction and desire to reproduce, this part of the brain can't distinguish the difference between people and images. Your subconscious believes you are in the middle of it.

Unable to distinguish the difference, the brain is trapped where reality and fantasy are inseparable, creating a hyper-sexualized worldview. A worldview that becomes more and more difficult to leave behind the longer you stay in it. When the addiction really takes hold, you might withdraw socially to enable your addiction. you might make your addiction into a routine. In extreme cases, you might become unable to participate in daily life without indulging in your addiction. Your brain has become rewired to satisfy your addiction.

How has porn affected your life? What have you skipped? How many restless nights? How many times have you passed on living your life? The time you and I had spent watching porn took years of our lives we can't get back.

Now you have two options: do nothing and waste your life, or do something about it.

A good start will be separating fantasy from reality and intentionally retraining the brain. This is not an easy or comfortable process, and it will require a lot of effort to rewire the neural processes you have trained.

The brain uses behaviors and habits like tools to diagnose and resolve issues. Whenever you feel a sexual urge, you open your toolbox and pull out whatever tools you have learned to use to solve your problem. In this case porn. This seems like it works, but over time you notice this tool isn't working -like using a butterknife instead of a screwdriver. Over time it becomes less effective, and you damage the screw as well.

And like the butterknife, porn is the wrong tool for the job. It hurts you whether you are aware or not. Each time you watch porn, you'll want more. But every time you resist porn, it gets easier. Take a deep breath, and let it pass. It will go away.

When we watch porn, under the surface level emotion of arousal is guilt. Any form of sexual immorality, regardless of what emotion drives the action, will inevitably be overshadowed by guilt. That guilt is a natural reaction to breaking our Moral Conscience, given to us by God.

> *"Deep within his conscience man discovers a law which he has not laid upon himself but which he must obey. Its voice, ever calling him to love and to do what is good and to avoid evil, sounds in his heart at the right moment... For man has in his heart a law inscribed by God... His conscience is man's most secret core and his sanctuary. There he is alone with God whose voice echoes in his depths" (Catechism of the Catholic Church[1]).*

And for those who want it straight from The Bible:

> *"But this is the new covenant which I will make with the house of Israel after those days, says the Lord: I will put my law within them, and I will write it upon their hearts; and I will be their God, and they shall be my people."*
>
> **Jeremiah 31:33**

In violating our Moral Conscience we feel the effects from sin, which separates us from our relationship with God. Sinning, with full awareness, intent, and in a significant matter, brings shame and guilt with it. This is why you picked up this book, why you are trying to be better. As you start to quit porn, you will learn what works for you.

Sometimes, it only takes something small to get rid of pornographic thoughts. In the beginning, I would shake

---

[1] Catholic Church., *Catechism of the Catholic Church.*

my head. It seems insignificant, but it is effective. Or take a second to get up and walk around. Or try the most effective thing I have found to work; pray. Prayer is the most powerful tool we have. It is a gift from God.

2

Rules, Tips 'n' Tricks

Some of you are thinking," I just want to quit porn, not be given rules to follow." But here's the cold hard truth, if you weren't struggling to quit porn you wouldn't have picked up this book. While I can't guarantee that these will work as well for you it is better than doing nothing.

Some people are more prone to addiction than others. The dopamine the brain releases when watching porn is powerful and highly addictive. Moreover, addiction is a self-destructive coping method. Maybe stress or neglect and porn numbed the loneliness. Everyone has their own story. Regardless of what got you into pornography, you want to climb out of it now, and it is a struggle. The first step to quit is prayer, the foundation of healing. Next, find the willpower to act it out. Without it, you'll be unprepared to resist temptation.

    This will require discipline and focus. Look at the top-performing athletes today and the amount of work they put in. They train their whole lives just for the opportunity to get recruited, and it doesn't even guarantee that they will go pro. They have to be in peak condition. They likely have strict diets and sleep routines to perform at their best. They follow rules and training programs diligently to be the best. And you have to, too. Start with rule #1, and when you have that under your belt pick up the next one. You are training yourself for success

1. Uphold Chastity

    Simply put no porn, masturbation, or fornication (sex out of marriage). Most porn addicts can't go more than three days without ejaculating, so this is the best place to start. This is a lifestyle change, not just breaking a habit. If you have tried this before, good. Try again. Use the other steps to make this a lifestyle change instead of breaking a habit. This will be uncomfortable and painful. But this is normal.

> *"More than that, we rejoice in our sufferings, knowing that suffering produces endurance, and endurance produces character, and character produces hope, and hope does not disappoint us, because God's love has been poured into our hearts through the Holy*

RULES, TIPS 'N' TRICKS

Spirit who has been given to us."

Romans 5:3-5

In our suffering, we develop endurance, to sustain prolonged suffering. In enduring suffering, we develop character, a moral fortitude that strengthens us. Through character, we start hoping and eventually develop peace. To get there we have to face our use of porn. If you are tempted, try these.

1. Think through the consequences, both physical and mental. Think about the shame that has loomed over you because of your porn consumption and how you live your life because of it. Think about what better things you could do instead. Think about the physical effects of porn: addiction, isolation, increased aggression, distorted views about relationships and sex, low self-esteem, neglect of aspects of their life, and Erectile Dysfunction which 18.4% of men in their 20s have, almost one out of every five guys.

2. Ask why you watch porn. Are you using it to reduce stress? Find a healthier outlet. Do you watch it because you feel lonely? Find a social group that is a good influence. Or are you tempted by lust? In that case, take a break to distance yourself from the temptation.

3. Break porn down for what it is. It's not an escape, it's a company that's out to make a profit. It is a formula- one improved upon since

the inception of porn. Even the soap opera-style acting, in the beginning, is intentional. After extended use, your brain is conditioned so that seeing this acting style flips a switch, creating arousal artificially in anticipation. In this sense, we are no better than Pavlov's dogs.

4. Have a strong motivation. It can be a lifestyle, it could be to grow closer to God, it could be to gain self-control of a crazy life. Everyone has their reason, but the important thing is to find a strong motivation where porn is the obstacle in your way. Personally, I imagine the life I want to build - a faith-based family. If you can't think of a goal, imagine your life without porn.

The best place to start taking the first step and building that future is to **uphold chastity**.

2. Don't Date for the First Three Months

Outside of yourself, porn harms others when relationships are involved. You think a good partner will motivate you to quit porn, However, relationships don't typically have any impact on reducing porn consumption, and likely any reduction that occurs is temporary. And this doesn't account for the obstacle porn is to creating a successful relationship. For starters, pursuing a woman with the primary goal of being sex is not substantially different from pornography and it can be argued that it is worse than porn because you are forcing an unwilling person to be your fantasy.

To be clear, this does not mean ending a serious relationship. If you are not in a serious relationship, are not dating with the intention of marriage, or are single, then this is for you. Don't date for the first three months. Use these three months to focus on humanizing people instead of objectifying them. Dating won't pull you away from porn. It's not supposed to. It would only set you back and hurt someone else. Instead, focus on developing genuine and healthy friendships and finding a healthy community, ideally one that is faith-based. Developing healthy friendships in healthy communities leads to healthy relationships. Then, when you finally meet the person you're going to marry, your future spouse won't suffer because you're watching porn.

If you are in a serious relationship but are not yet married, avoid sleeping with your partner. Commit to abstinence until you are married. Be honest with your partner. Tell them what you are facing and that you don't want it to affect your relationship going forward. If they want to spend the rest of their life with you, they'll be supportive or happy that you are putting effort into your future together. It will get difficult for you both, and you might mess up. But get through this together, and you will be much closer as a couple.

Some think that if you have already had sex, it won't make any difference if you practice chastity. That it can't get worse, but it can. We all have made mistakes, and way back then, people made the same mistakes we make today. Take Romans 13:12-14:

> *"The night is far gone, the day is at hand. Let us then cast off the works of darkness and put on the armor of light; let us conduct ourselves becomingly as in the day, not in reveling and drunkenness, not in debauchery and licentiousness, not in quarreling and jealously. But put on the Lord Jesus Christ, and make no provision for the flesh, to gratify its desires."*

Our mistakes and sins are the whole reason Jesus came down in the first place, not only to pardon our transgressions but to set an example of how we should live our lives.

If you are married, you aren't exempt from this rule. Tell them you are quitting porn and desire to give them your full attention romantically. Take them out on dates. Intentionally pursue the woman you chose above all women, not a pixelated lady who doesn't even know you exist. Focus on your spouse selflessly.

If your spouse doesn't know about your relationship with porn, tell them. This will not be an easy conversation, but it is important. You need to hold yourself accountable and will need their support. They will not be happy with you, but you need to reset your relationship and build it on a firm foundation.

Make it clear that you love your spouse. I don't mean to tell them, show them. Date them like you used to. Don't initiate sex. Make it clear to your spouse what you are trying to do and give them the power to initiate sex. Focus on deepening your emotional relationship with them instead. Must be clear that you don't see them as a sex object, which creates more resentment and marriage issues. The most important thing is to put visible effort into loving your spouse. **Stay dedicated to your recommitment to date your spouse and not use porn to meet your desires.** Marriage is a beautiful thing, a sacred institution given by God. Chastity is the best way to honor the gift of marriage. To clarify sex isn't a bad thing, but your spouse is more important than pleasure.

If you think watching porn doesn't impact your marriage, you're wrong. Statistically speaking, exposure to pornography doubles the odds of divorce for men and triples the odds for women and is a leading cause of divorce. The top two reasons for divorce are lack of commitment and infidelity/extramarital affairs. Porn contributes to both. If you want to take that risk, be my guest but your decision will affect much more than you and your spouse.

For the rest of you who aren't married or in a relationship, **don't date for the first three months.**

3. Men, Have a Meal Plan

In 2016, a study was published examining the behavioral and psychological relationships between sex and eating.[2] In men, there is a correlation between the desire for food and the desire for sex. Not only that, they found that men with a high desire for food also have a high desire for sex. This study noted that women do not have the same correlation between sex and food as men do. So this rule is for men only.

Since the same part of the brain is active when men want either food or sex, then learning to be disciplined in what we eat will also discipline us in how we deal with sexual desire. Be disciplined—not on a diet.

Eat real food; eat salty and sugary foods in moderation. Don't eat when you're not hungry. When you start to snack, decide if you are actually hungry or if you are bored. Portion your food to what you need. If you feel like snacking, drink water or chew gum for 30 minutes before you decide if you are hungry enough to eat.

If you want a basic example, this is a simple meal plan I used:

Eat a big breakfast, do not eat carbs after 3 pm, and eat just meat and vegetables for dinner around 6 pm. A more religious meal plan would include supplementing meat (except fish) on Fridays.

[2] Kang, Zheng, and Zheng, "Sex and Eating."

You don't have to follow the same meal plan I did, make one that works for you. It could be as simple as no junk food or soda, or as complicated as tracking macros with intermediate fasting. The important thing is to be intentional with what you eat. **Have a meal plan.**

4. Have an Exercise Routine

When upholding chastity you will notice several things. In as early as one week, others will start to notice too - specifically friends often notice an excess of energy. I have seen guys, after just a week, have seemingly limitless energy, becoming hyperactive and hyper-social. From that point, the urges will come suddenly, forcefully, and unexpectedly. In repelling those impulses, people become easily irritable and lash out more.

When upholding chastity you will notice several things. In as early as one week, others will start to notice too—specifically friends often notice an excess of energy. I have seen guys, after just a week, have seemingly limitless energy, becoming hyperactive and hyper-social. From that point, the urges will come suddenly, forcefully, and unexpectedly. In repelling those impulses, people become easily irritable and lash out more.

Developing an exercise routine will build mental strength, help repel the desire for porn, and also retrain the brain with coping stress or anxiety. In developing an exercise routine, your brain will jump to exercise instead of pornography to de-stress and even burn off some excess energy you don't know what to do with.

It doesn't have to be an intense workout. The point is to teach yourself healthy ways to manage stress while dealing with your pent-up energy. **Have an exercise routine.**

5. Set up roadblocks

Everyone has a "ritual" before they watch porn, actions they take to prepare for it. For some, it's grabbing tissues and lube. Others a gross sock. Others have a specific time and place to watch porn. Become aware of your habits. Take steps to make them difficult.

Maybe you watch porn while lying in bed at night. If so, charge your phone in a separate room. Maybe you use a sock, if so, throw it away. Maybe you use tissues and lube. If so, throw them out, and don't re-buy them.

Make it difficult to access pornography. Install a website blocker on your phone and computer, turn on safe search on your search engine so they won't pop up, and turn on parental controls on your phone. Limit how long you are on social media. If you see something that makes you want to watch porn, block the post, and leave the app. If you don't watch porn even once, it's working. Congratulate yourself. But if you can't remove the temptation, then remove yourself from the situation. Walking away is often more effective than trying to face it head-on. **Set up roadblocks.**

6. Find your community

Who you spend time with will affect every aspect of your life. If you are with successful people, you will become more successful; if you are with faithful people, you will grow in faith. It also works the other way; if you are with lazy people, you will become lazy; if you are around faithless people, you will act faithlessly. On the topic at hand, if you surround yourself with people who see nothing wrong with porn, hookups, etc. then inevitably, you will behave that way.

Unfortunately, sex and pornography are cultural norms today. Many people, secular and Christian alike, contribute to normalizing it, intentionally or not. This is why community is so important. Surround yourself with people who acknowledge that porn and sex outside of marriage are self-destructive. Find an accountability partner for when you feel pulled to porn or sex. While I didn't have an accountability partner, I have been for someone else, and it's an effective tool.

On the flip side, observe the lives of people who go out of their way to hook up or settle for porn when they can't. Are they happy? Are they living their life like a happy person would? Do not judge them, but notice if they are truly, genuinely happy. And I don't mean how it looks on social media. Are they happy in their day-to-day life? Are they living their life like someone happy would?

I found with most people who were focused on getting laid, whenever the possibility of sex arose, they became focused on interacting with sex as the end goal. Porn is the same way, it can overpower every thought.

Some Christians downplay being sexually promiscuous and watching pornography. Ask them why, and they will brush it off. Some will say that since Jesus died for our sins and will always forgive our sins, that sinning is inconsequential. But Paul states:

> *"What Then? Are we to sin because we are not under law but under grace? By no means! Do you not know that if you yield yourselves to any one as obedient slaves, you are slaves of the one whom you obey, either to sin, which leads to death, or of obedience, which leads to righteousness?"*
> **Romans 8:15-16**

While we all fall short and sin, and while Jesus did die for and forgive us of our sins if we ask, we do not have a free pass to do whatever we want. There are still consequences to sin. It still separates us from God and leads us to commit more serious sins and to sin more frequently.

Everyone has people you know deep down you should spend less time with, and other people that you don't hang around enough, but you know you should. What happens when you are around people you shouldn't be around? You do things you shouldn't do. What happens when you hang with those you should hang around? You do good things you wouldn't have done on your own. When you hang out with a group of people, what is important to most of the group is important to all of you. It's human nature.

So in the pursuit of quitting porn, you will need people who don't watch porn or who are walking away from it as well. **Find your Community.**

7. Break the Fantasy

In 1995, Doskoch found that on average, men will have seven sexual fantasies a day, while women will have four and a half fantasies a day.[3] In 2020 The US did a national survey and found that 68.4% of adolescents have seen porn.[4] In the same year, a US study was released saying 42% of kids 10-17 have viewed porn. The 26% not accounted for are likely outside the age demographic—in other words, under 10 years old.[5] How will they grow up to see the world? Will it be a fantasy to them? Or will they be unable to see the world in any way other than sexually? Every person they find attractive will be a temptation for them to see as only a compilation of body parts, not as the

---

[3] Miranda and Medeiros, "The Normality of Sexual Fantasies."
[4] Jhe et al., "Pornography Use among Adolescents and the Role of Primary Care."
[5] Ibid.

individual God created them to be.

These are real people. The people who imagine their sexual fantasies usually use people they know or see in real life. They use these people, playing a role in their sexual fantasies, to fill that void of desire. Fantasies can come in many forms—a desire they would never want to admit to. A self-medication to isolation or low self-worth, the problem is sexual fantasies are one-dimensional and self-serving perceptions of relationships. They tend to regress into dark and violent fantasies over time to overcome the high tolerance of dopamine.

Sexual fantasies and pornography are synonymous. The only difference is the level of control you have. Fantasies are more personal; you're the one creating the fantasy. But they are still one-dimensional at best. The person in that fantasy is not the person you saw, and you aren't yourself in the fantasy either. Fantasy blends pornography and the world around you. These fantasies are about self-gratification and sex instead of a relationship, which is self-sacrificial in nature.

Fantasies are easy. There is little effort and no risk of rejection. As you embrace fantasy, you pull away from genuine, tangible, and real relationships, making it more difficult to build true and healthy relationships now and in the future.

So, to develop healthy relationships, start with the

basics. Relationships are built with mutual respect and values, not on sexual gratification - and the ones that are don't last. Fantasies separate us from these possible relationships through objectification. In fantasizing, you deny the reality of who that person is, leaving both parties hurt. One falls in love with a figment of their imagination, only to be disappointed when the other person ends up nothing like the fantasy. The other wants to be loved for who they are, only to be heartbroken by realizing that the other person didn't like them for anything expect their body. If you want a genuine and healthy relationship, leave behind the fantasy and live in reality.

As it says in 1 Thessalonians 4: 3-8, we are supposed to be self-disciplined and capable of controlling ourselves and our actions. Are we going to get it right every time? Probably not. We are all imperfect and broken individuals. But that doesn't mean we shouldn't try.

Let's say I have a bow, two arrows, and a target 50 feet away. I shoot the first arrow. I might hit the target, but I might not. I might only hit the target once a month, missing the shot every other day. But even when I miss, the first arrow is closer than the arrow I never shot. But the more I shoot, the better I will get, and the more often I will hit the mark. The only way I'll improve is by trying.

It is the same way with resisting pornography. Some people you fantasize about may not be anyone other than someone you saw walking down the street last Tuesday.

Others you probably see every day.

Start with the people you are closest to that you fantasize about. When you notice yourself in a fantasy, shut down the fantasy. Reinforce the break with facts about how it isn't real. Remind yourself that they are people and look for what makes them unique as a person instead of what makes you want them to be a 2-D fantasy.

Next are the people you see frequently but don't know. It could be a classmate you know but have never spoken with or someone you see at the gym frequently. Start by talking to them. it can be as simple as, "Hey, I see you here all the time, but I don't think I've ever actually met you." From there, just have a simple and short conversation, not to gain anything from it or with any end goal in mind, but to learn about them. You might be surprised by how interesting people can be. Even if you don't find them interesting, now you have a baseline impression of that person. Now, they are not strangers but someone you know, a friend with feelings and dreams.

In doing so, you have broken the fantasy by humanizing them, by seeing the person they are instead of a physical body to lust over. Eventually, the idea of fantasizing, in general, will feel wrong and perverse.

Another way to dissolve a fantasy of someone is to associate them as someone you would never fantasize about. If they are around your age, associate them with someone you are unattracted to. Trying to see them as family members instead of associating them with a typical porn trope is usually the simplest.

In humanizing these people you fantasize about, not only are you keeping yourself firmly planted in reality, which is a necessity in quitting porn, but also in developing stronger and healthier relationships as a whole. You will learn to see people as they are instead of who you imagine them to be, and you will appreciate them more than the fantasy you've imagined. So, when building healthy relationships, leave behind your sexual fantasies and **break the fantasy.**

8. Do What is Good

Once, when I was in confession, I was confessing how I fell into lust, and the priest gave me some wisdom I'm passing down to you. He said that instead of white knuckling my way through hardships, focusing on what not to do, I should focus on what to do. Essentially: do what is good. Instead of telling yourself not to watch porn, replace that with what you should do. Have you done something to deepen your faith? Have you done something else that you can do? Something you want to try?

Leaving porn and living a chaste life does not happen overnight. It will take time - at least months, but possibly years. Even if it takes years, isn't it better than a life of shame? Live a life not of justifying the actions you know are wrong, but of choosing to pursue what is right. **Do what is good.**

9. Pray

I brushed off prayer for a long time. Sure, I believed prayer helped people, and I had no problem praying for others. However, I didn't feel the same way about myself. I thought porn was something I needed to face, something to overcome myself. Prayer wouldn't help that, could it? And when I tried on my own, I failed over and over again, never seeing a single breakthrough.

During the COVID lockdowns, when I decided to change what I could change, I was already miserable. Since I was already miserable, adding on abstinence would be easy. It didn't last a day. I tried again and failed again. It wasn't until I found my reason why I wanted to quit that I could abstain. And with all the willpower I could muster, it only bought me eight months.

Those eight months were very grueling and formative months of my life. I started on the path that led to me becoming Catholic. After I relapsed, I decided to research how porn affects the brain and addictions as a whole. It reduced my porn consumption significantly, but it still wasn't zero. I was able to live a close-to-abstinent life for a while until a new year. I Drank too much at a party. You can guess the rest.

RULES, TIPS 'N' TRICKS

After this, I despaired. The despair was consuming me. So I did something new and, as a non-Catholic, went to confession. Since I was in faith formation, I was allowed to participate in confession. I opened up everything that I did, and after being pardoned, it felt as if a gentle light pierced into my head and pulled off the despair. I prayed to God, asking him to remove the temptation of porn from me, but it didn't work that way. I was still tempted. Then, as I was sitting in adoration, pondering my struggle with lust, a thought crossed my mind.

What if I'm not meant to defeat lust? Instead, I'm supposed to leave this to Jesus. So I started praying. I told Jesus I tried everything in my power and couldn't do it, but that I knew He could, that I submit to His will.

I didn't feel a spiritual awakening, and I didn't feel anything special happening. But I started again, this time pursuing chastity instead of abstinence. This time, I noticed I was less tempted, and it was easier to overcome. Whenever I faced temptation, I'd pray an Our Father, which helped.

"Our Father, Who art in heaven, Hallowed be Thy Name. Thy Kingdom come. Thy Will be done, on earth as it is in Heaven. Give us this day our daily bread. And forgive us our trespasses, as we forgive those who trespass against us. And lead us not into temptation, but deliver us from evil. Amen."

I'm not saying you'll never face temptation again. Jesus faced temptation. But praying and asking for help with temptation is much easier than trying to do it with your power.

It's not a "pray once and all your problems will go away" situation. It's not a magical cure-all. God will help and strengthen you, but He will not do it for you. Your active participation is required as well. You have to be deliberate. If you believe God is who He says He is trust in Him and **pray.**

The Blueprint

When starting, it is a good idea to install web blocks and have someone you trust put parental controls on your app store. Focus on what you should do not what you shouldn't. Follow the rules and their core principles:

1. **Uphold Chastity**- no sex outside of marriage; practice abstinence.

2. **Don't Date for the First Three Months**- Being in a relationship won't solve your problems and could hurt you or someone else.

3. **Have a Meal Plan**- Build your self-discipline and your self-control.

4. **Have an Exercise Routine**- Burn off your excess energy healthily and productively.

RULES, TIPS 'N' TRICKS

5. **Set Up Roadblocks-** Make it difficult for yourself to access pornography.

6. **Find Your Community-** Surround yourself with healthy people who live the way you want to live.

7. **Break the Fantasy-** Ground yourself in reality and humanize those you fantasize about.

8. **Do What is Good-** Prioritize what you should be doing instead of what you are avoiding.

9. **Pray-** Ask for God's intervention and allow him to act for you.

3

What to Expect

Quitting porn will cause you to experience many discomforts, which vary from person to person, comes and goes in waves, and doesn't happen all at once—at least it didn't for me.

Increased Irritability

You got a temper before you quit porn? Yeah, it will get worse before it gets better. Assuming it improves at all. When abstaining, your brain isn't producing as much dopamine as before. Because of that, your brain has to reset. To your new normal expect to feel irritable for a couple of weeks. The best way to work through this is exercising. For men, a meal plan.

Intensified Anxiety

Having anxiety can mean anything from having intense, pessimistic, and possibly unrealistic fears about potential outcomes to being overwhelmed by too many options. As you abstain, you will likely experience periods of intensified anxiety. But remember this:

> *"Therefore I tell you, do not be anxious about your life, what you shall eat or what you shall drink, nor about your body, what you shall put on. Is not life more than food, and the body more than clothing? Look at the birds of the air: they neither sow nor reap nor gather into barns, and yet the heavenly father feeds them. Are you not of more value than they? And which of you by being anxious can add one cubit to his span of life?"*
>
> **Matthew 6:25-27**

I'm not saying to ignore problems or to not think ahead, but when you're anxious, pray. Tell God what you are going through and leave it at His feet, trusting His plan. Stressing about it won't help.

> *"But seek first his kingdom and his righteousness, and all these things shall be yours as well. Therefore do not be anxious about tomorrow, for tomorrow will be anxious for itself. Let the day's own trouble*

be sufficient for the day."
Matthew 6:33-34

Depression

Yes, depression can be a symptom you will experience. Don't stress over it. It's due to dopamine withdrawals your brain hasn't yet adjusted. Having a healthy community will help you work through it. It will fade away on its own. Avoiding fantasies and dating without intention will help it pass by more quickly. If you are concerned or suicidal, seek professional help. Asking for help doesn't make you weak, it's accepting you need help. And it takes a strong person to acknowledge when they need help and to seek it.

Brain Fog

It's safe to assume by now you have already experienced this from porn. And the difference in brain fog from watching porn and from abstaining is minimal. Brain fog that comes from consuming porn is mostly due to dehydration. Brain fog from abstinence is more due to hormonal imbalance. It comes and goes. Having a daily routine worked wonders for me. Over time, the brain adjusts to routines and expects the routine. If you relapse, reduce the brain fog by drinking 2-3 glasses of water. This will rehydrate you and reduce the brain fog, helping you get on track. Forcing yourself to think, read, write, and other mental activities will help reduce brain fog.

Emotional Numbness

This is more obscure, but don't underestimate this. If you do, you will relapse without knowing what went wrong. After you get through this phase—for me a couple of months—you'll experience stronger emotions than before, and it will take time to adjust. You'll begin to feel you're taking your life back. At this point, you'll begin to understand what you lost because of porn.

Porn Cravings

This is self-explanatory. If you deprive yourself of any addiction, you will crave it. Prayer is vital here. I used the "Our Father" prayer to get through this. I'd repeat the prayer until the urge subsided or I could repress it. These cravings will most likely hit when you are in a situation you have previously. Either fantasized or given into the temptation of porn. The majority of the rules aimed at reducing this, especially #7.

Loss of Libido

This isn't necessarily a bad thing, in you aren't as likely to watch porn, but it does give a false sense of victory.

Eventually, you might think something is wrong since you're not experiencing arousal. Don't worry, everything works. I went through this and relapsed because I thought something was wrong and decided to self-evaluate. But nothing was wrong, and I had to start over from square one. If you experience this, learn from my mistakes, and let it run its course.

Porn Flashes

Have you ever watched war movies where it shows the soldiers after they get back from the war and they'll have PTSD flashbacks? You're going to go through the porn equivalent of it. Nowhere near as traumatizing, but it's still not pleasant. At first, these will happen all the time with every sound, sight, or thought remotely associated with porn. Over time, they will fade away. Just don't ruminate and let yourself get absorbed by them. The best way to ground yourself is through prayer.

Lack of Sleep

For me, this was the worst obstacle to overcome. Nobody likes waking up in the middle of the night feeling like their privates are on fire, too aroused to go back to bed. At first, it was unbearable and constant, and it was a toss-up of what I'd do. At one point, I tried staying awake reading or working to keep my mind off it, but I wouldn't recommend that solution. For me, sleep deprivation does not make any of this easier. This phase started about four to six weeks in. And lasted for months. The longest consecutive span with interrupted sleep was about 10 days. It wasn't until a friend at my church recommended praying the rosary before sleeping that I was able to make any progress in overcoming this obstacle. I didn't have a rosary or know how to pray one. But my friend gave me a rosary and instructions on how to pray it as well. I went home, prayed the rosary, and slept for the first time in months.

I am eternally grateful to Mary for interceding for my rest. While you could pray anything before sleeping, try praying the rosary once.

Porn Dreams

Most likely, if you started watching porn before puberty, you didn't have wet dreams or did very rarely. You thought you lucked out, but not quite. When you quit porn, there is a chance you'll have these types of dreams. Other than being embarrassing, this shouldn't be an issue at all. If you wake up to a mess, don't stress over it and clean it up. Then go back to sleep.

The Ugly Truth

On paper, these effects sound bad, and this process sounds uncomfortable, which it is uncomfortable. But it's temporary. What's a few months, or even a year, of discomfort to a lifetime of peace, free from the constraints of porn and sexual immorality?

God has your best interest at heart. Everything He does is for your good, and here, in pursuing righteousness, God will give you what you need. Paul states our weakness is an opportunity for God to work in us. That His power is perfect within our faults. Not an excuse for our weakness but a comfort for our inadequacies.

> *"And to keep me from being too elated by the abundance of revelations, a thorn was given me in the flesh, a messenger of Satan, to harass me, to keep me from being too elated. Three times I begged the Lord about this, that it should leave me; but he said to me, 'My grace is sufficient for you, for my power is made perfect in weakness.'"*
> **2 Corinthians 12:7-8**

What You'll Face Outside of Withdrawals

It wouldn't feel right to talk about what you face when quitting pornography and not talk about this. As you pursue chastity and draw closer to God you will also find things will try to get in your way. Seemingly ordinary obstacles timed conveniently to stop your progress. Or maybe they will come across as something entirely different.

When I was quitting porn, it was always when I felt like I had made it, that I experienced the most temptation or my lowest relapse. This might happen to you as well.

When I started writing this book, I began to experience vivid porn flashes, so vivid I'd close the computer and walk away. I faced that every time I wrote for a month. After I was able to shake off the porn flashes, I started receiving pornographic emails in my spam folder. Yes, I go through my spam folder. So, I did what any person would do and deleted it. The next time I went through my email, I saw another one. And another one. I emptied the whole spam folder - I didn't want another temptation, especially while writing this book. The next time I checked, over half my spam folder was porn related. I couldn't figure out why I was getting these. I never used my actual email, always fake emails, and deleted those emails whenever I quit. I didn't want to see these spam emails; I looked to see if I could block them, but I couldn't. I noticed one of the emails was a hookup site. The email made it look like I had an account on it. I clicked the link, and an account was already made. Horrified, I found the account management page and deleted the account. I returned to five more emails. Each is from a different hookup site. I did the same to those - then 10 new emails, all to different sites. I unsubscribed and immediately got another email from a nearly identical site. Later, I checked my email and saw 137 spam emails since the afternoon. All of them were pornographic. I was

WHAT TO EXPECT

even starting to get emails that weren't flagged as spam that were porn related. I got fed up and decided to delete them here and there but not to stress over it. I still get about 50-100 porn emails daily.

You might find yourself being the subject of other people's desires, founded on their lust. Giving into those temptations will not do well for you. It won't do for you what you think it will, and you won't feel fulfilled after; you'll feel emptier.

You might start experiencing unrelated things that will make you want porn or take a break from chastity. You could be put in a position where you previously failed, in hopes that you will make the same mistake again. After, you could beat yourself up with guilt to the point you give up. Remember that the source of any addiction is pain and regret. After my email fiasco and a few temptations I encountered, I started having other problems. I started arguing with my family, and after that was resolved, I had to put down my dog. These problems happened relentlessly, consistently, one after the other.

Life happens, and when we choose to follow Jesus, we encounter problems. Fortunately, Jesus also shows us how to face these occurrences.

> *"And the tempter came and said to him,*
> *'If you are the Son of God, command these*
> *stones to become loaves of bread.'*

> *But he answered, 'It is written, "Man shall not live by bread alone, but by every word that proceeds from the mouth of God"'*
>
> **Matthew 4: 3-4**

Focus on Him above your problems. When Peter walked on water it was only because of Jesus that it was possible, but by keeping his eyes on Jesus he was able to do something remarkable and impossible. Keep your eyes on Jesus because as soon as you look away, like Peter, you will start to sink.

Epilogue

When facing pornography or any sexual immorality, we often feel we are powerless against our temptations. One day we are on top; the next at rock bottom. If we try to overcome it with our strength, we'll fail. Even if you succeed, you missed the whole point. Rely on an inexhaustible strength. One that can't tire or be beaten. Compared to that level of strength, our burden is light.

After quitting porn, life has been much more peaceful. I wouldn't say easy, but peaceful. Relationships are more impactful and built on mutual respect instead of mutual desires. I fervently hope this book will be a trusty guide as you strive to live the Christian life away from the lures of pornography and fornication.

Reread this book when you struggle to help find a solution, but also take the time to orient yourself properly, submitting yourself to God and His Will. All these tools are helpful, but God is the best physician. He can cure any ailment, solve any problem, and even better, He knows the exact remedy for you.

"But Jesus looked at them and said to them, "With men this is impossible, but with God all things are possible."
Matthew 19:26

Bibliography

Catholic Church. *Catechism of the Catholic Church: Modifications from the Editio Typica.* Vatican: Libreria Editrice Vaticana, 1997.

Jhe, Grace B, Jessica Addison, Jessica Lin, and Emily Pluhar. "Pornography Use among Adolescents and the Role of Primary Care." *Family Medicine and Community Health* 11, no. 1 (January 2023): e001776. https://doi.org/10.1136/fmch-2022-001776.

Kang, Ying, Lijun Zheng, and Yong Zheng. "Sex and Eating: Relationships Based on Wanting and Liking." *Frontiers in Psychology* 6 (January 11, 2016). https://doi.org/10.3389/fpsyg.2015.02044.

Miranda, Kristin, and Alisha Medeiros. "The Normality of Sexual Fantasies." *California State University, Stanislaus*, 2005. https://www.csustan.edu/sites/default/files/honors/documents/journals/sexinstone/Miranda&Medeiros.pdf.

Milton Keynes UK
Ingram Content Group UK Ltd.
UKHW030944220724
445981UK00014B/708